The Ultimate Ket e
Colle

CW00456109

Delicious Mouth-watering R
He

Tia Graham

Table of contents

3

Basil Zucchinis and Eggplants

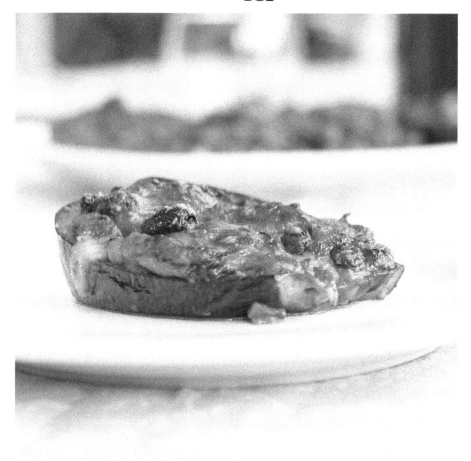

Preparation time: 10 minutes Cooking time: 20 minutes Servings: 4

Ingredients:

1 tablespoon olive oil

2 zucchinis, sliced

1 eggplant, roughly cubed

2 scallions, chopped

1 tablespoon sweet paprika

Juice of 1 lime

1 teaspoon fennel seeds, crushed

Salt and black pepper to the taste

1 tablespoon basil, chopped

Directions:

1. Heat up a pan with the oil over medium heat, add the scallions and fennel seeds and sauté for 5 minutes.

2. Add zucchinis, eggplant and the other ingredients, toss, cook over medium heat for 15 minutes more, divide between plates and serve as a side dish.

Nutrition: calories 97, fat 4, fiber 2, carbs 6, protein 2

Chard and Peppers Mix

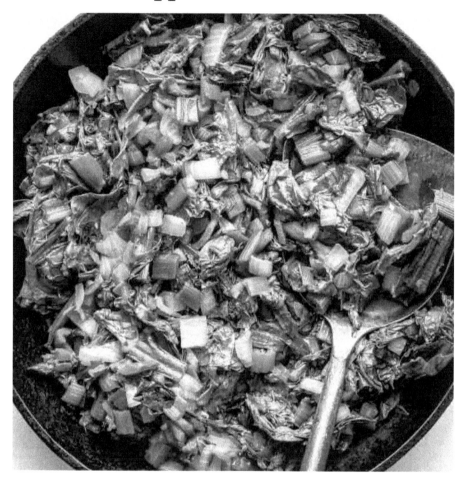

Preparation time: 10 minutes Cooking time: 20 minutes Servings: 4

Ingredients:

2   tablespoons avocado oil

2 spring onions, chopped

2 tablespoons tomato passata

2 tablespoons capers, drained

2 green bell peppers, cut into strips

1 teaspoon turmeric powder

A pinch of cayenne pepper

Juice of 1 lime

Salt and black pepper to the taste

1 bunch red chard, torn

Directions:

1.   Heat up a pan with the oil over medium heat, add the spring onions, capers, turmeric and cayenne and sauté for 5 minutes.

2.   Add the peppers, chard and the other ingredients, toss, cook over medium heat for 15 minutes more, divide between plates and serve.

Nutrition: calories 119, fat 7, fiber 3, carbs 7, protein 2

Balsamic Kale

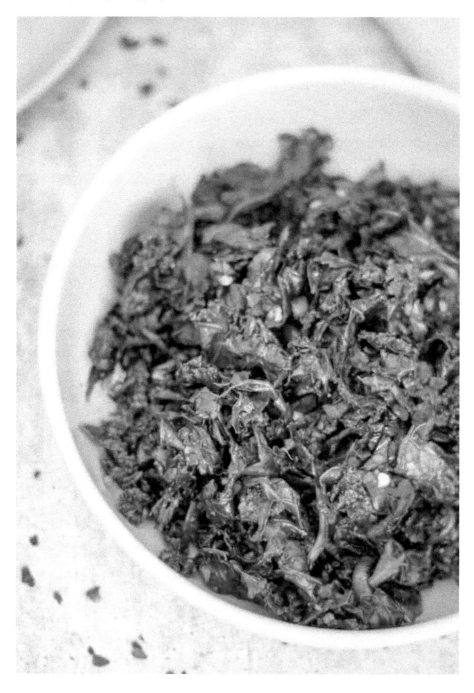

Preparation time: 10 minutes Cooking time: 20 minutes Servings: 4

Ingredients:

1 tablespoon balsamic vinegar

2 tablespoons walnuts, chopped

1 pound kale, torn

1 tablespoon olive oil

1 teaspoon cumin, ground

1 teaspoon chili powder

3 garlic cloves, minced

2 tablespoons cilantro, chopped

Directions:

1.   Heat up a pan with the oil over medium heat, add the garlic and the walnuts and cook for 2 minutes.

2.   Add the kale, vinegar and the other ingredients, toss, cook over medium heat for 18 minutes more, divide between plates and serve as a side.

Nutrition: calories 170, fat 11, fiber 3, carbs 7, protein 7

Mustard Cabbage Salad

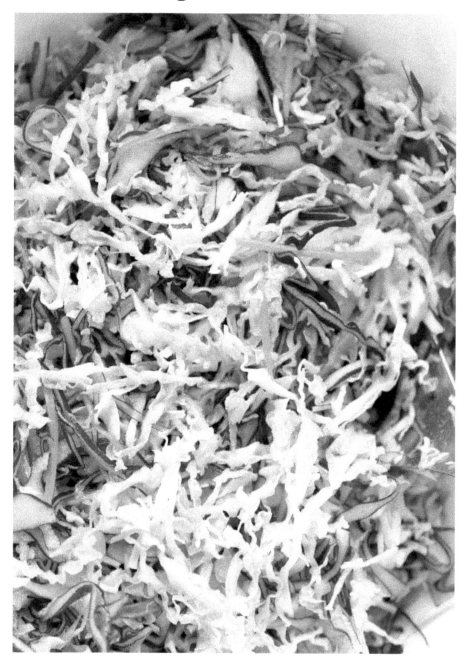

Preparation time: 10 minutes Cooking time: 0 minutes Servings: 4

Ingredients:

1   green cabbage head, shredded

1 red cabbage head, shredded

2   tablespoons avocado oil

2 tablespoons mustard

1 tablespoon balsamic vinegar

1 teaspoon hot paprika

Salt and black pepper to the taste

1 tablespoon dill, chopped

Directions:

1. In a bowl, mix the cabbage with the oil, mustard and the other ingredients, toss, divide between plates and serve as a side salad.

Nutrition: calories 150, fat 3, fiber 2, carbs 2, protein 7

Cabbage and Green Beans

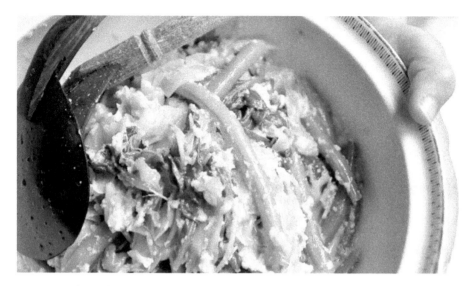

Preparation time: 10 minutes Cooking time: 15 minutes Servings: 4

Ingredients:

1   green cabbage head, shredded

2   cups green beans, trimmed and halved

2 tablespoons olive oil

1 teaspoon sweet paprika 1 teaspoon cumin, ground

Salt and black pepper to the taste

1 tablespoon chives, chopped

Directions:

1.   Heat up a pan with the oil over medium heat, add the cabbage and the paprika and sauté for 2 minutes.

2.   Add the green beans and the other ingredients, toss, cook over medium heat fro 13 minutes more, divide between plates and serve.

Nutrition: calories 200, fat 4, fiber 2, carbs 3, protein 7

Green Beans, Avocado and Scallions

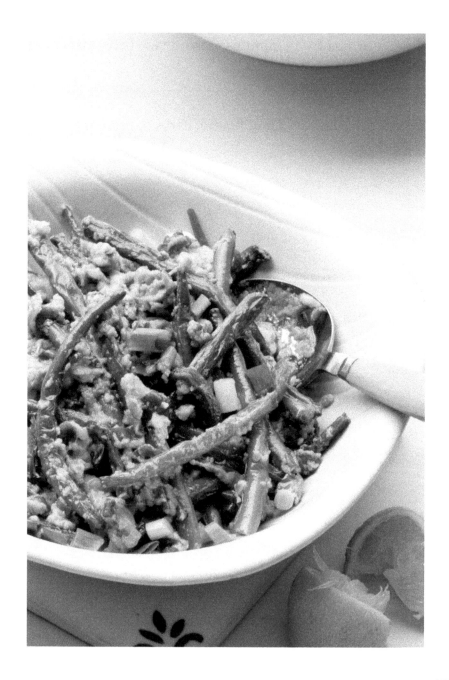

Preparation time: 10 minutes Cooking time: 20 minutes Servings: 4

Ingredients:

1 pound green beans, trimmed and halved

1 avocado, peeled, pitted and sliced

4 scallions, chopped

2 tablespoons olive oil

1 tablespoon lime juice

Salt and black pepper to the taste

A handful cilantro, chopped

Directions:

1.   Heat up a pan with the oil over medium heat, add the scallions and sauté for 2 minutes.

2.   Add the green beans, lime juice and the other ingredients, toss, cook over medium heat for 18 minutes, divide between plates and serve.

Nutrition: calories 200, fat 5, fiber 2,3, carbs 1, protein 3

Creamy Cajun Zucchinis

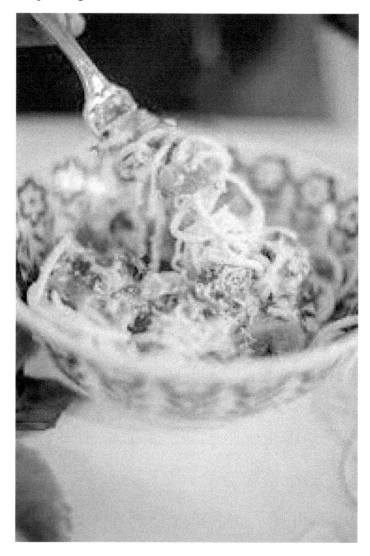

Preparation time: 10 minutes Cooking time: 20 minutes

Servings: 4

Ingredients:

1 pound zucchinis, roughly cubed

2 tablespoons olive oil

4 scallions, chopped

Salt and black pepper to the taste

1 teaspoon Cajun seasoning

A pinch of cayenne pepper

1 cup coconut cream

1 tablespoon dill, chopped

Directions:

1.   Heat up a pan with the oil over medium heat, add the scallions, cayenne and Cajun seasoning, stir and sauté for 5 minutes.

2.   Add the zucchinis and the other ingredients, toss, cook over medium heat for 15 minutes more, divide between plates and serve.

Nutrition: calories 200, fat 2, fiber 1, carbs 5, protein 8

Herbed Zucchinis and Olives

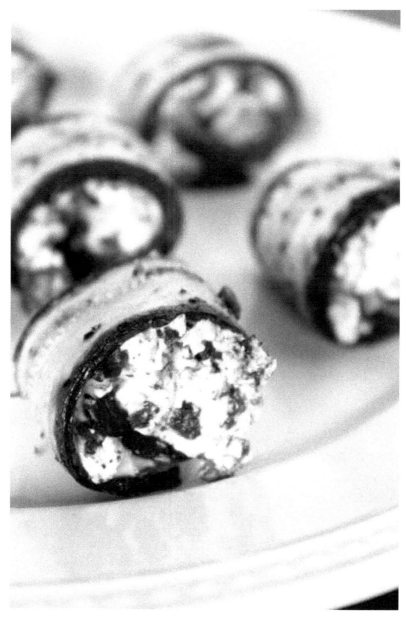

Preparation time: 10 minutes Cooking time: 20 minutes Servings: 4

Ingredients:

1 cup kalamata olives, pitted

1 cup green olives, pitted

1 pound zucchinis, roughly cubed

1 tablespoon rosemary, chopped

1 tablespoon basil, chopped

1 tablespoon cilantro, chopped

2 tablespoons olive oil

3 garlic cloves, minced

1 tablespoon lemon juice

1   teaspoon lemon zest, grated

1 tablespoon sweet paprika

A pinch of salt and black pepper

Directions:

1.   Heat up a pan with the oil over medium heat, add the garlic, lemon zest and paprika and sauté for 2 minutes.

2.   Add the olives, zucchinis and the other ingredients, toss, cook over medium heat for 18 minutes more, divide between plates and serve.

Nutrition: calories 200, fat 20, fiber 4, carbs 3, protein 1

Veggie Pan

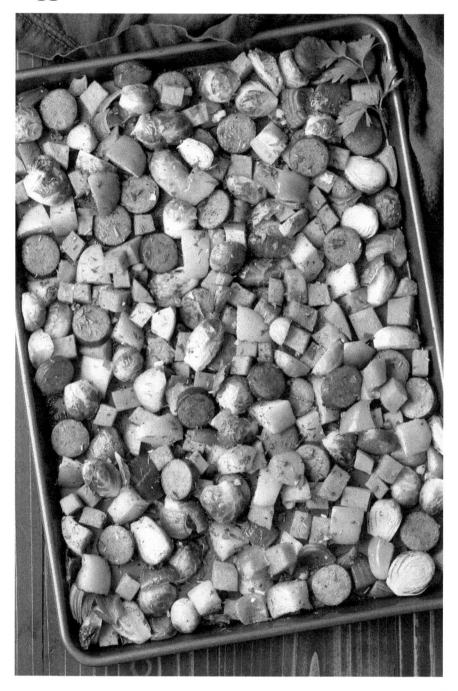

Preparation time: 10 minutes Cooking time: 20 minutes Servings: 4

Ingredients:

1 cup green beans, trimmed and halved

1 cup cherry tomatoes, halved

1 zucchini, roughly cubed

1 red bell pepper, cut into strips

1 eggplant, cubed

3 scallions, chopped

2 tablespoons olive oil

2 tablespoons lime juice

Salt and black pepper to the taste

1 teaspoon chili powder

1 tablespoon cilantro, chopped

3 garlic cloves, minced

Directions:

1.   Heat up a pan with the oil over medium heat, add the scallions, chili powder and the garlic and sauté for 5 minutes.

2.   Add the green beans, tomatoes and the other ingredients, toss, cook over medium heat for 15 minutes.

3.   Divide the mix between plates and serve as a side dish.

Nutrition: calories 137, fat 7.7, fiber 7.1, carbs 18.1, protein 3.4

Masala Brussels Sprouts

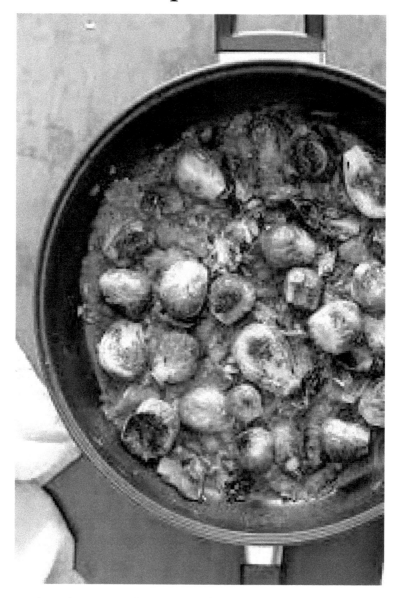

Preparation time: 10 minutes Cooking time: 35 minutes

Servings: 4

Ingredients:

1 pound Brussels sprouts, trimmed and halved

Salt and black pepper to the taste

1 tablespoon garam masala

2   tablespoons olive oil

1 tablespoon caraway seeds

Directions:

1.   In a roasting pan, combine the sprouts with the masala and the other ingredients, toss and bake at 400 degrees F for 35 minutes.

2.   Divide the mix between plates and serve.

Nutrition: calories 115, fat 7.6, fiber 4.9, carbs 11.2, protein 4.2

Nutmeg Green Beans

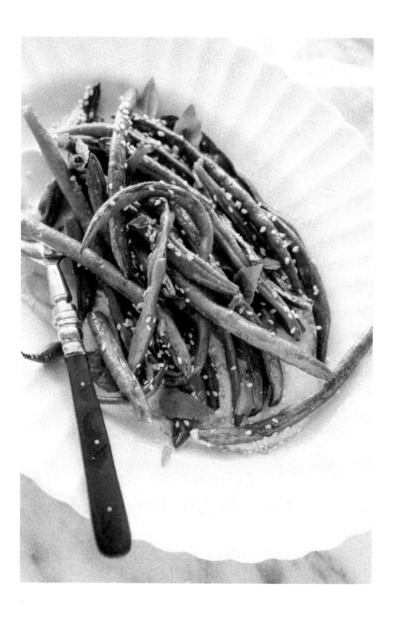

Preparation time: 10 minutes Cooking time: 30 minutes
Servings: 4

Ingredients:

2 tablespoons olive oil

½ cup coconut cream

1-pound green beans, trimmed and halved

1 teaspoon nutmeg, ground

A pinch of salt and cayenne pepper

½ teaspoon onion powder

½ teaspoon garlic powder

2   tablespoons parsley, chopped

Directions

1.   Heat up a pan with the oil over medium heat, add the green
beans, nutmeg and the other ingredients, toss, cook for 30
minutes, divide the mix between plates and serve.

Nutrition: calories 100, fat 13, fiber 2.3, carbs 5.1, protein 2

Peppers and Celery Sauté

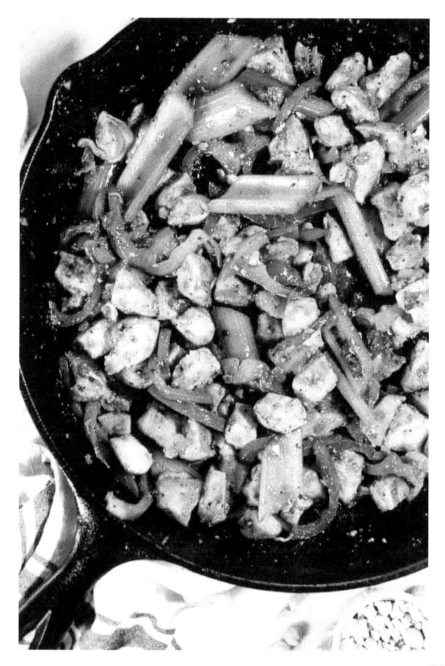

Preparation time: 10 minutes Cooking time: 15 minutes

Servings: 4

Ingredients:

1 red bell pepper, cut into medium chunks

1   green bell pepper, cut into medium chunks

1 celery stalk, chopped

2   scallions, chopped

2 tablespoons olive oil

Salt and black pepper to the taste

1 tablespoons parsley, chopped

1 teaspoon cumin, ground

2 garlic cloves, minced

Directions:

1.   Heat up a pan with the oil over medium heat, add the scallions, garlic and cumin and sauté for 5 minutes.

2.   Add the peppers, celery and the other ingredients, toss, cook over medium heat for 10 minutes more, divide between plates and serve.

Nutrition: calories 87, fat 2.4, fiber 3, carbs 5, protein 4

Oregano Zucchinis and Broccoli

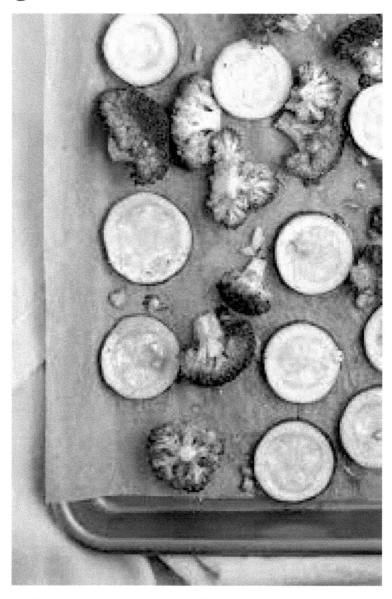

Preparation time: 10 minutes Cooking time: 20 minutes Servings: 4

Ingredients:

1-pound zucchinis, sliced

1 cup broccoli florets

Salt and black pepper to the taste

2 tablespoons avocado oil

2   tablespoons chili powder

½ teaspoon oregano, dried

1 and ½ tablespoons coriander, chopped

Directions:

1.   Heat up a pan with the oil over medium heat, add the zucchinis, broccoli and the other ingredients, toss, cook over medium heat for 20 minutes, divide between plates and serve as a side dish.

Nutrition: calories 140, fat 2, fiber 1, carbs 1, protein 6

Spinach Mash

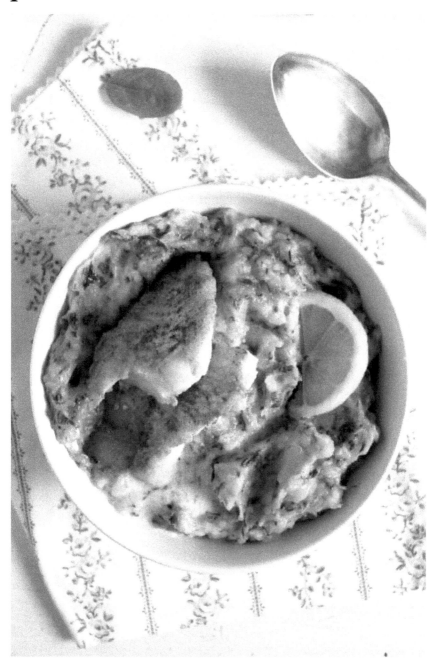

Preparation time: 10 minutes Cooking time: 15 minutes Servings: 4

Ingredients:

1   pound spinach leaves

3 scallions, chopped

2   garlic cloves, minced

¼ cup coconut cream

2 tablespoons olive oil

Salt and black pepper to the taste

½ tablespoon chives, chopped

Directions:

1.   Heat up a pan with the oil over medium heat, add the scallions and the garlic and sauté for 2 minutes.

2.   Add the spinach and the other ingredients except the chives, toss, cook over medium heat for 13 minutes, blend using an immersion blender, divide between plates, sprinkle the chives on top and serve.

Nutrition: calories 190, fat 16, fiber 7, carbs 3, protein 5

Jalapeno Zucchinis Mix

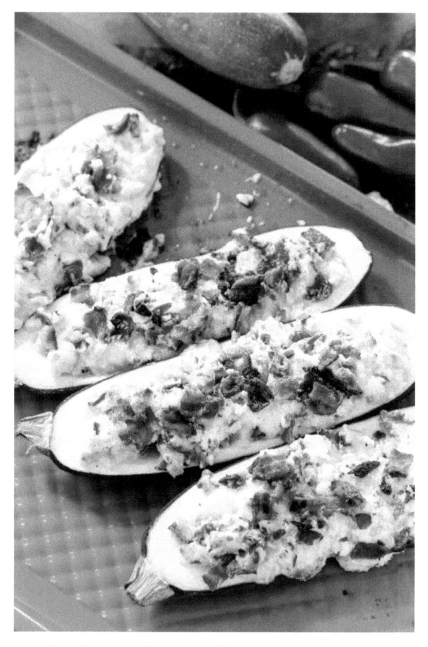

Preparation time: 10 minutes Cooking time: 30 minutes Servings: 4

Ingredients:

1 pound zucchinis, sliced

¼ cup green onions, chopped

½ cup cashew cheese, shredded

1 cup coconut cream

2   jalapenos, chopped

Salt and black pepper to the taste

2 tablespoons chives, chopped

Directions:

1.   In a baking dish, combine the zucchinis with the onions and the other ingredients, toss, bake at 390 degrees F for 30 minutes, divide between plates and serve.

Nutrition: calories 120, fat 4.2, fiber 2.3, carbs 3, protein 6

Coconut and Tomatoes Mix

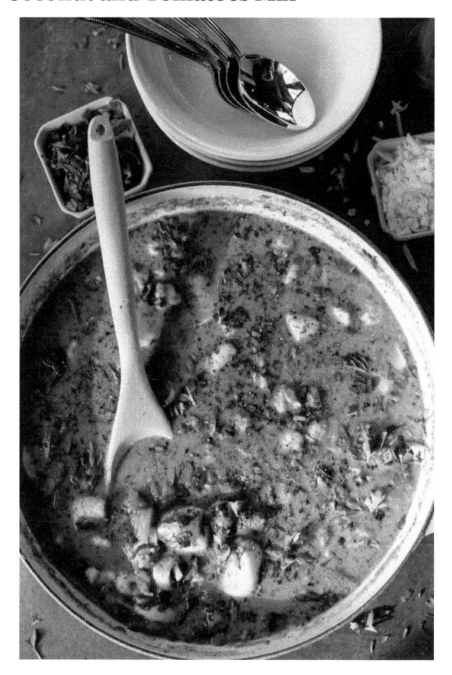

Preparation time: 5 minutes Cooking time: 12 minutes Servings: 4

Ingredients:

1 pound tomatoes, cut into wedges

1 cup coconut, unsweetened and shredded

2 tablespoons coconut oil, melted

1   tablespoon chives, chopped

1 teaspoon coriander, ground

1 teaspoon fennel seeds

Salt and black pepper to the taste

Directions:

1.   Heat up a pan with the oil over medium heat, add the coriander and fennel seeds and cook for 2 minutes.

2.   Add the tomatoes and the other ingredients, toss, cook over medium heat for 10 minutes, divide between plates and serve.

Nutrition: calories 152, fat 13.8, fiber 3.4, carbs 7.7, protein 1.8

Mushroom Rice

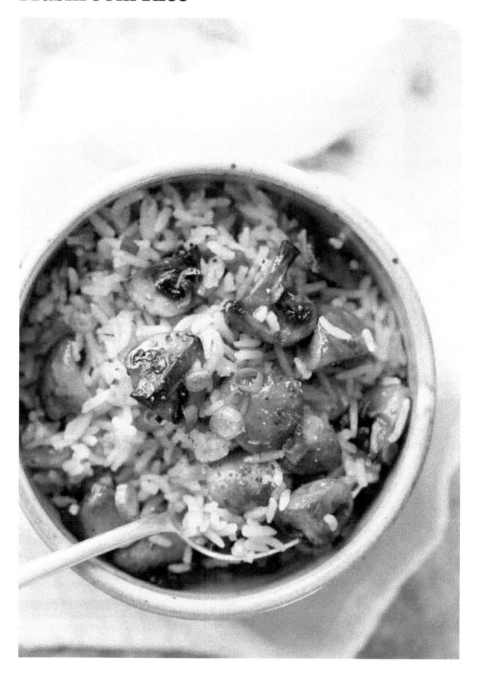

Preparation time: 10 minutes Cooking time: 20 minutes Servings: 4

Ingredients:

2   tablespoons olive oil

1   cup mushrooms, sliced

2 cups cauliflower rice

2   tablespoons lime juice

2 tablespoons almonds, sliced

1 cup veggie stock

Salt and black pepper to the taste

½ teaspoon garlic powder

1 tablespoon parsley, chopped

Directions:

1.   Heat up a pan with the oil over medium heat, add the mushrooms and the almonds and sauté for 5 minutes.

2.   Add the cauliflower rice and the other ingredients, toss, cook over medium heat for 15 minutes more, divide between plates and serve.

Nutrition: calories 124, fat 2.4, fiber 1.5, carbs 2, protein 1.2

Cucumber and Cauliflower Mix

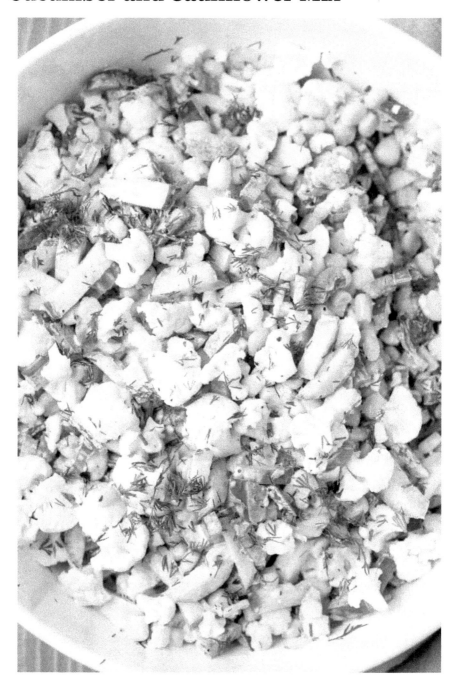

Preparation time: 10 minutes Cooking time: 12 minutes Servings: 4

Ingredients:

1 cucumber, cubed

1   pound cauliflower florets

1 spring onion, chopped

2   tablespoons avocado oil

1 tablespoon balsamic vinegar

¼ teaspoon red pepper flakes

Salt and black pepper to the taste

1 tablespoon thyme, chopped

Directions:

1.   Heat up a pan with the oil over medium heat, add the spring onions and the pepper flakes and sauté for 2 minutes.

2.   Add the cucumber and the other ingredients, toss, cook over medium heat for 10 minutes more, divide between plates and serve.

Nutrition: calories 53, fat 1.2, fiber 3.9, carbs 9.9, protein 3

Mushroom and Spinach Mix

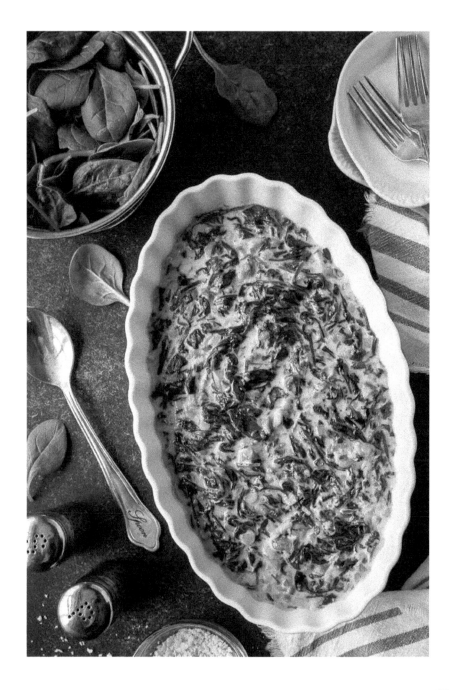

Preparation time: 10 minutes Cooking time: 15 minutes Servings: 4

Ingredients:

1 cup white mushrooms, sliced

3 cups baby spinach

2 tablespoons olive oil

Salt and black pepper to the taste

2 tablespoons garlic, minced

2 tablespoons pine nuts, toasted

1 tablespoon walnuts, chopped

Directions:

1. Heat up a pan with the oil over medium heat, add the garlic, pine nuts and the walnuts and cook for 5 minutes.

2. Add the mushrooms and the other ingredients, toss, cook over medium heat for 10 minutes, divide between plates and serve.

Nutrition: calories 116, fat 11.3, fiber 1.1, carbs 3.5, protein 2.5

Garlic Cauliflower Rice

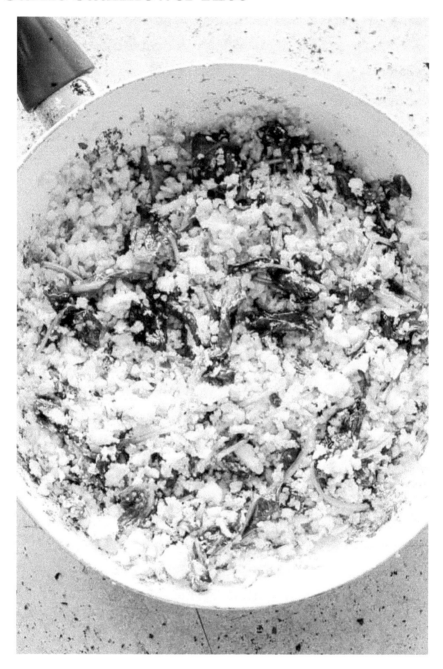

Preparation time: 10 minutes Cooking time: 20 minutes Servings: 4

Ingredients:

2 cups cauliflower rice

2 tablespoons almonds, chopped

1 tablespoon olive oil

2   green onions, chopped

4 garlic cloves, minced

3   tablespoons chives, chopped

½ cup vegetable stock

Directions:

1.   Heat up a pan with the oil over medium heat, add the garlic and green onions and sauté for 5 minutes.

2.   Add the cauliflower rice and the other ingredients, toss, cook over medium heat for 15 minutes, divide between plates and serve.

Nutrition: calories 142, fat 6.1, fiber 1.2, carbs 3, protein 1.2

Grapes and Tomato Salad

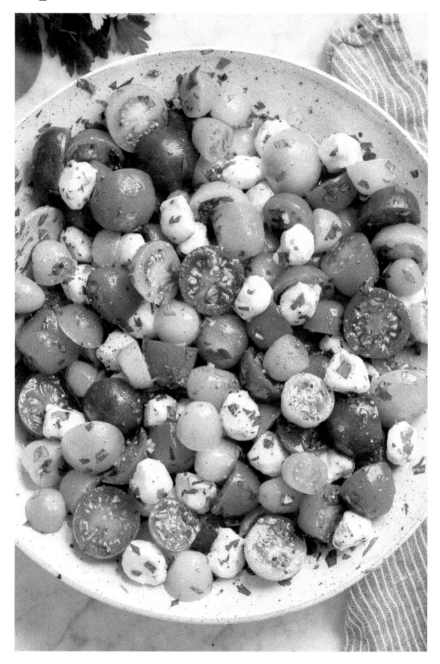

Preparation time: 10 minutes Cooking time: 0 minutes Servings: 4

Ingredients:

2 cups green grapes, halved

1 pound cherry tomatoes, halved

2 tablespoons olive oil

4 spring onions, chopped

1 teaspoon cumin, ground

1 teaspoon rosemary, dried

1 tablespoon balsamic vinegar

1 tablespoon chives, chopped

Directions:

1.   In a bowl, combine the grapes with the tomatoes and the other ingredients, toss and serve as a side salad.

Nutrition: calories 140, fat 4, fiber 6, carbs 3.4, protein 4

Tomato and Walnuts Vinaigrette

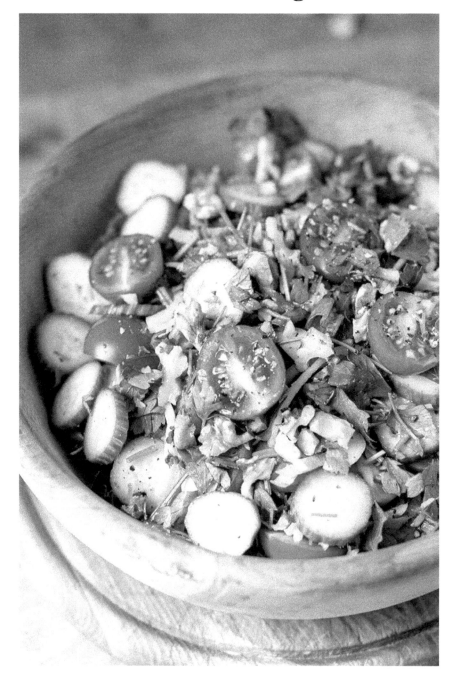

Preparation time: 10 minutes Cooking time: 0 minutes Serving: 4

Ingredients:

1 pound cherry tomatoes, halved

1 tablespoon walnuts, chopped

1 tablespoon balsamic vinegar

1   garlic clove, minced

1 teaspoon lemon juice

2   teaspoons smoked paprika

¼ teaspoon coriander, ground

Salt and black pepper to the taste

1 tablespoon parsley, chopped

Directions:

1.   In a bowl, combine the tomatoes with the walnuts and the other ingredients, toss well, and serve as a side dish.

Nutrition: calories 160, fat 12, fiber 4, carbs 6, protein 4

Creamy Eggplant Mix

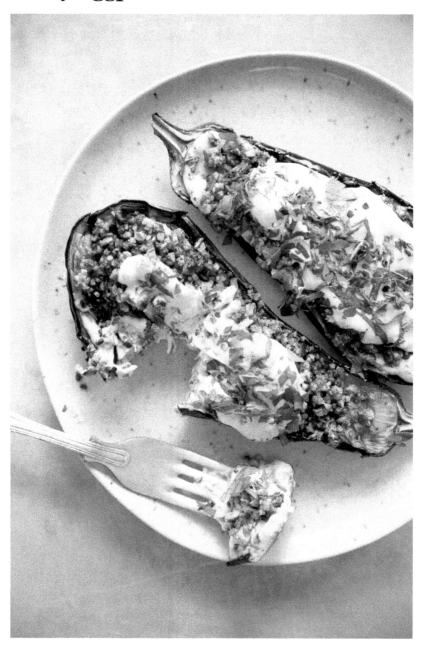

Preparation time: 10 minutes Cooking time: 15 minutes Servings: 4

Ingredients:

1 pound eggplants, roughly cubed

2 scallions, chopped

2   tablespoon avocado oil

2 teaspoons garlic, minced

½ cup coconut cream

2 teaspoons chili paste

Directions:

1.   Heat up a pan with the oil over medium heat, add the scallions and the garlic and sauté for 2 minutes.

2.   Add the eggplants and the other ingredients, toss, cook over medium heat for 13 minutes more, divide between plates and serve as a side dish.

Nutrition: calories 142, fat 7, fiber 4, carbs 5, protein 3

Chives Kale and Tomato

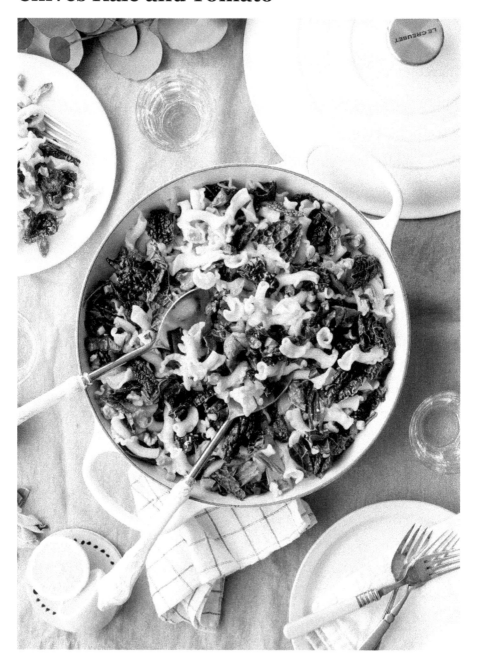

Preparation time: 10 minutes Cooking time: 20 minutes Servings: 4

Ingredients:

1 pound kale, torn

½ pound tomatoes, cut into wedges

2 tablespoons avocado oil

1 teaspoon chili powder

1 teaspoon garam masala

Salt and black pepper to the taste

¼ teaspoon coriander, ground

A pinch of cayenne pepper

1 teaspoon mustard powder

¼ cup chives, chopped

Directions:

1.   In a roasting pan, combine the kale with the tomatoes and the other ingredients, toss and bake at 380 degrees F for 20 minutes.

2.   Divide the mix between plates and serve as a side dish.

Nutrition: calories 128, fat 2.3, fiber 1, carbs 3.3, protein 4

Cauliflower Salad

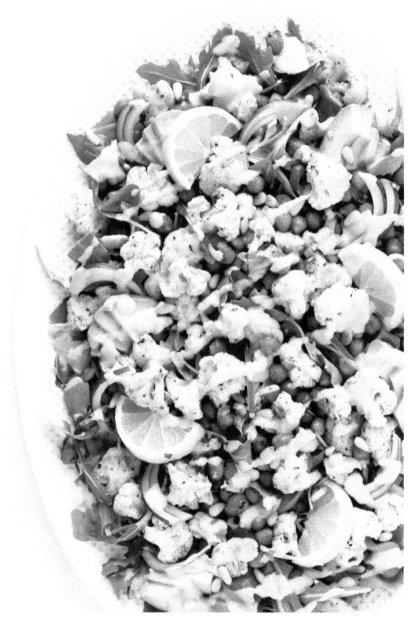

Preparation time: 10 minutes Cooking time: 0 minutes Servings: 4

Ingredients:

1 pound cauliflower florets, blanched

1 avocado, peeled, pitted and cubed

1 cup kalamata olives, pitted and halved

Salt and black pepper to the taste

1 cup spring onions, chopped

1 tablespoon lime juice

1 tablespoon chives, chopped

Directions:

1.   In a bowl, combine the cauliflower florets with the avocado and the other ingredients, toss and serve as a side salad.

Nutrition: calories 211, fat 20, fiber 2, carbs 3, protein 4

Turmeric Carrots

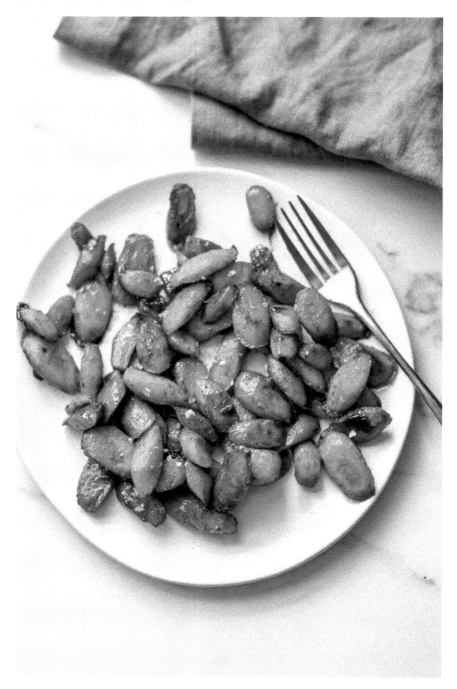

Preparation time: 10 minutes Cooking time: 40 minutes Servings: 4

Ingredients:

1   pound baby carrots, peeled

1 tablespoon olive oil

2   spring onions, chopped

2 tablespoons balsamic vinegar

2 garlic cloves, minced

1 teaspoon turmeric powder

1 tablespoon chives, chopped

¼ teaspoon cayenne pepper

A pinch of salt and black pepper

Directions:

1.   Spread the carrots on a baking sheet lined with parchment paper, add the oil, the spring onions and the other ingredients, toss and bake at 380 degrees F for 40 minutes.

2.   Divide the carrots between plates and serve.

Nutrition: calories 79, fat 3.8, fiber 3.7, carbs 10.9, protein 1

Spinach Mix

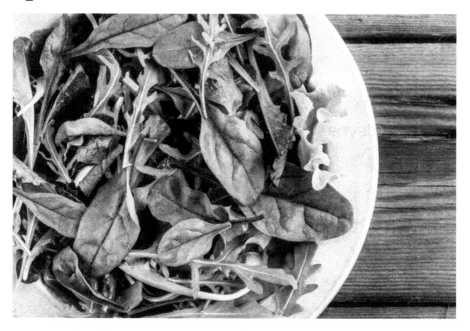

Preparation time: 10 minutes Cooking time: 12 minutes Servings: 4

Ingredients:

1 pound baby spinach

1 yellow onion, chopped

1 tablespoon olive oil

1 tablespoon lemon juice

2 garlic cloves, minced

A pinch of cayenne pepper

¼ teaspoon smoked paprika

A pinch of salt and black pepper

Directions:

1.   Heat up a pan with the oil over medium-high heat, add the onion and the garlic and sauté for 2 minutes.

2.   Add the spinach and the other ingredients, toss, cook over medium heat for 10 minutes, divide between plates and serve as a side dish.

Nutrition: calories 71, fat 4, fiber 3.2, carbs 7.4, protein 3.7

Orange Carrots

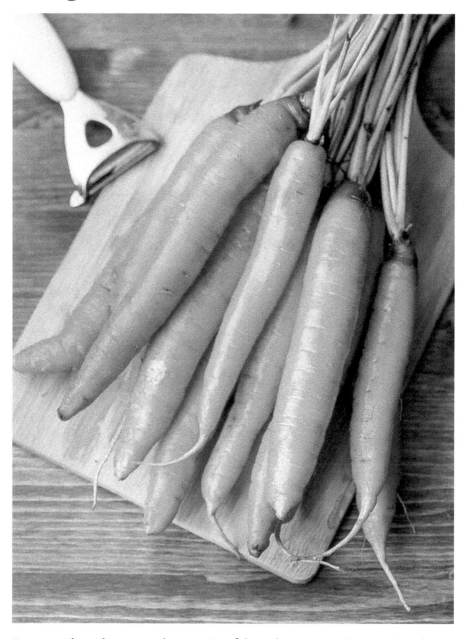

Preparation time: 5 minutes Cooking time: 25 minutes Servings: 4

Ingredients:

1 pound carrots, peeled and roughly sliced

1 yellow onion, chopped

1 tablespoon olive oil

Zest of 1 orange, grated

Juice of 1 orange

1 orange, peeled and cut into segments

1 tablespoon rosemary, chopped

A pinch of salt and black pepper

Directions:

1.   Heat up a pan with the oil over medium-high heat, add the onion and sauté for 5 minutes.

2.   Add the carrots, the orange zest and the other ingredients, toss, cook over medium heat for 20 minutes more, divide between plates and serve.

Nutrition: calories 140, fat 3.9, fiber 5, carbs 26.1, protein 2.1

Endive Sauté

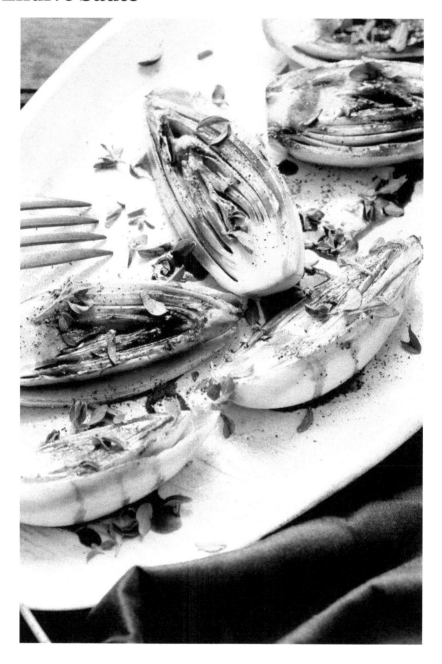

Preparation time: 5 minutes Cooking time: 15 minutes Servings: 4

Ingredients:

3 endives, shredded

1 tablespoon olive oil

4 scallions, chopped

½ cup tomato sauce

2 garlic cloves, minced

A pinch of sea salt and black pepper

1/8 teaspoon turmeric powder

1 tablespoon chives, chopped

Directions:

1.   Heat up a pan with the oil over medium heat, add the scallions and the garlic and sauté for 5 minutes.

2.   Add the endives and the other ingredients, toss, cook everything for 10 minutes more, divide between plates and serve as a side dish.

Nutrition: calories 110, fat 4.4, fiber 12.8, carbs 16.2, protein 5.6

Zucchini Pan

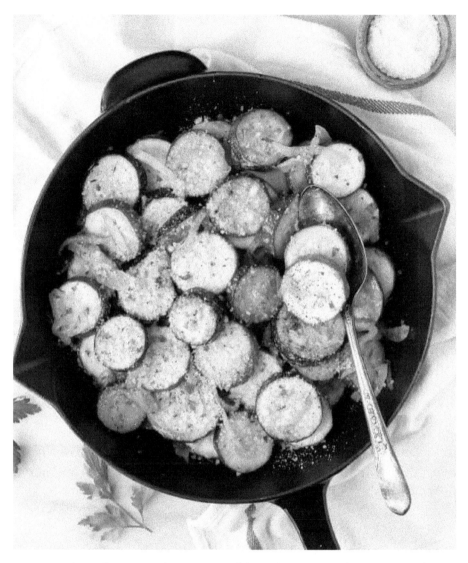

Preparation time: 5 minutes Cooking time: 20 minutes Servings: 4

Ingredients:

1 pound zucchinis, sliced

1 yellow onion, chopped

2 tablespoons olive oil

2   apples, peeled, cored and cubed

1 tomato, cubed

1 tablespoon rosemary, chopped

1 tablespoon chives, chopped

Directions:

1.   Heat up a pan with the oil over medium heat, add the onion and sauté for 5 minutes.

2.   Add the zucchinis and the other ingredients, toss, cook over medium heat for 15 minutes more, divide between plates and serve as a side dish.

Nutrition: calories 170, fat 5, fiber 2, carbs 11, protein 7

Ginger Mushrooms

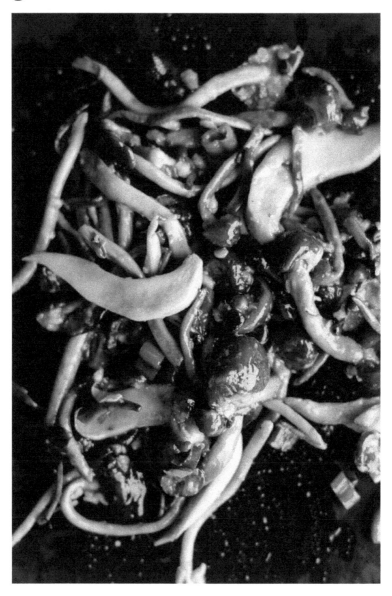

Preparation time: 10 minutes Cooking time: 20 minutes Servings: 4

Ingredients:

1 pound mushrooms, sliced

1 yellow onion, chopped

1   tablespoon ginger, grated

1 tablespoon olive oil

2   tablespoons balsamic vinegar

2 garlic cloves, minced

A pinch of salt and black pepper

¼ cup lime juice

2 tablespoons walnuts, chopped

Directions:

1.   Heat up a pan with the oil over medium-high heat, add the onion and the ginger and sauté for 5 minutes.

2.   Add the mushrooms and the other ingredients, toss, cook over medium heat for 15 minutes more, divide between plates and serve.

Nutrition: calories 120, fat 2, fiber 2, carbs 4, protein 5

Bell Pepper Sauté

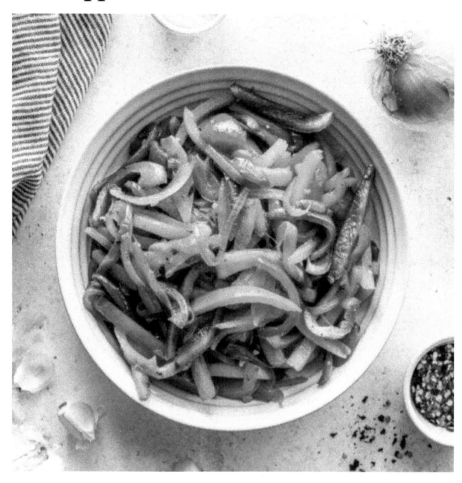

Preparation time: 5 minutes Cooking time: 20 minutes Servings: 4

Ingredients:

1 red bell pepper, cut into strips

1 yellow bell pepper, cut into strips

1 green bell pepper, cut into strips

1 orange bell pepper, cut into strips

3 scallions, chopped

1 tablespoon olive oil

1 tablespoon coconut aminos

A pinch of salt and black pepper

1 tablespoon parsley, chopped

1 tablespoon rosemary, chopped

Directions:

1.   Heat up a pan with the oil over medium-high heat, add the scallions and sauté for 5 minutes.

2.   Add the bell peppers and the other ingredients, toss, cook over medium heat for 15 minutes more, divide between plates and serve.

Nutrition: calories 120, fat 1, fiber 2, carbs 7, protein 6

Kale and Tomatoes

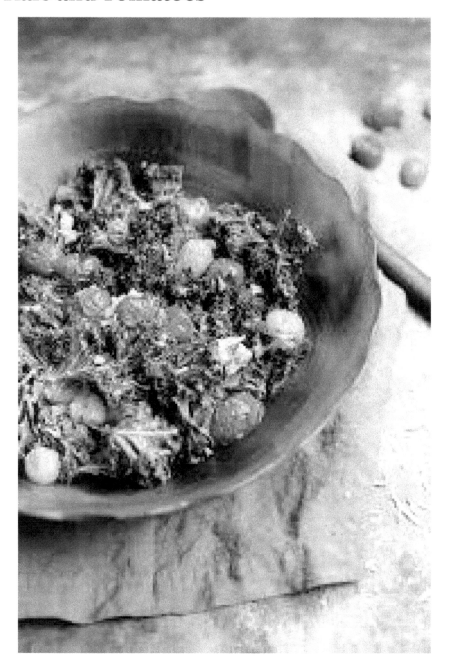

Preparation time: 5 minutes Cooking time: 20 minutes Servings: 4

Ingredients:

1 cup cherry tomatoes, halved

1 pound baby kale

1 yellow onion, chopped

2 tablespoons olive oil

1 tablespoon balsamic vinegar

1 tablespoon cilantro, chopped

2 tablespoons vegetable stock

A pinch of salt and black pepper

Directions:

1.   Heat up a pan with the oil over medium heat, add the onion and sauté for 5 minutes.

2.   Add the kale, tomatoes and the other ingredients, toss, cook over medium heat for 15 minutes more, divide between plates and serve as a side dish.

Nutrition: calories 170, fat 6, fiber 6, carbs 9, protein 4

Chili Artichokes

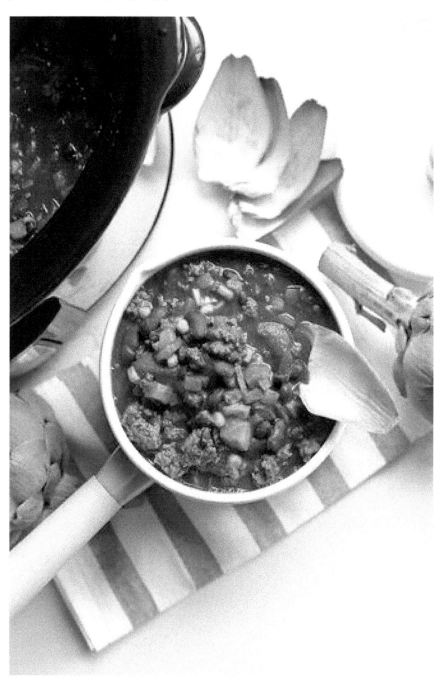

Preparation time: 10 minutes Cooking time: 25 minutes Servings: 4

Ingredients:

2 artichokes, trimmed and halved

1 teaspoon chili powder

2 green chilies, mined

2 tablespoons olive oil

1   teaspoon garlic powder

1 teaspoon sweet paprika

A pinch of salt and black pepper

Juice of 1 lime

Directions:

1.   In a roasting pan, combine the artichokes with the chili powder, the chilies and the other ingredients, toss and bake at 380 degrees F for 25 minutes.

2.   Divide the artichokes between plates and serve.

Nutrition: calories 132, fat 2, fiber 2, carbs 4, protein 6

Brussels Sprouts Mix

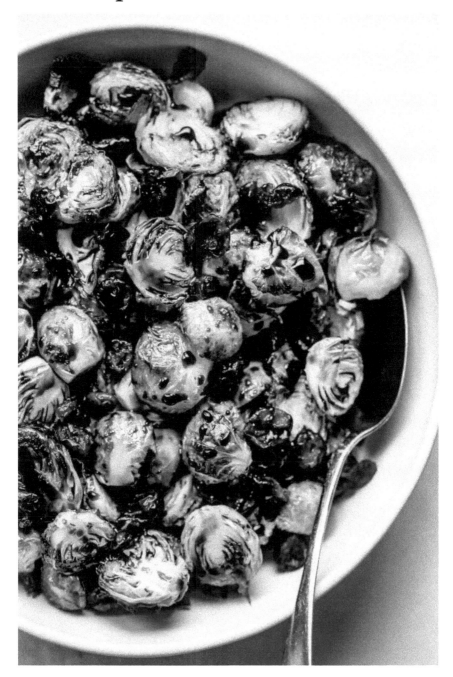

Preparation time: 10 minutes Cooking time: 20 minutes Servings: 4

Ingredients:

2 tablespoons olive oil

1 pound Brussels sprouts, trimmed and halved

1 tablespoon ginger, grated

2 garlic cloves, minced

1 tablespoon pine nuts

1 tablespoon olive oil

Directions:

1.   Heat up a pan with the oil over medium heat, add the garlic and the ginger and sauté for 2 minutes.

2.   Add the Brussels sprouts and the other ingredients, toss, cook for 18 minutes more, divide between plates and serve.

Nutrition: calories 160, fat 2, fiber 2, carbs 4, protein 5

Cauliflower Mix

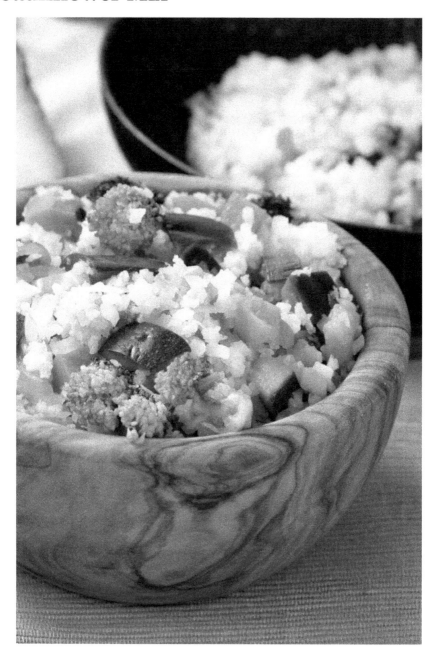

Preparation time: 10 minutes Cooking time: 25 minutes Servings: 4

Ingredients:

1 pound cauliflower florets

2 tablespoons avocado oil

1 teaspoon nutmeg, ground

1 teaspoon hot paprika

1 tablespoon pumpkin seeds

1 tablespoon chives, chopped

A pinch of sea salt and black pepper

Directions:

1.   Spread the cauliflower florets on a baking sheet lined with parchment paper, add the oil, the nutmeg and the other ingredients, toss and bake at 380 degrees F for 25 minutes.

2.   Divide the cauliflower mix between plates and serve as a side dish.

Nutrition: calories 160, fat 3, fiber 2, carbs 9, protein 4

Baked Broccoli and Pine Nuts

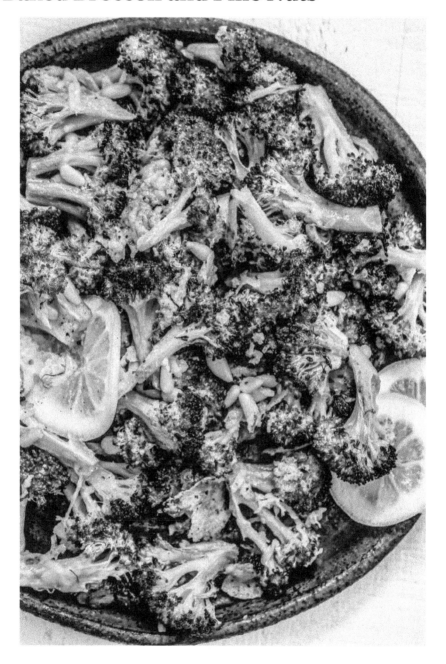

Preparation time: 10 minutes Cooking time: 30 minutes Servings: 4

Ingredients:

2   tablespoons olive oil

1 pound broccoli florets

1 tablespoon garlic, minced

1   tablespoon pine nuts, toasted

1 tablespoon lemon juice

2   teaspoons mustard

A pinch of salt and black pepper

Directions:

1.   In a roasting pan, combine the broccoli with the oil, the garlic and the other ingredients, toss and bake at 380 degrees F for 30 minutes.

2.   Divide everything between plates and serve as a side dish.

Nutrition: calories 220, fat 6, fiber 2, carbs 7, protein 6

Quinoa and Peas

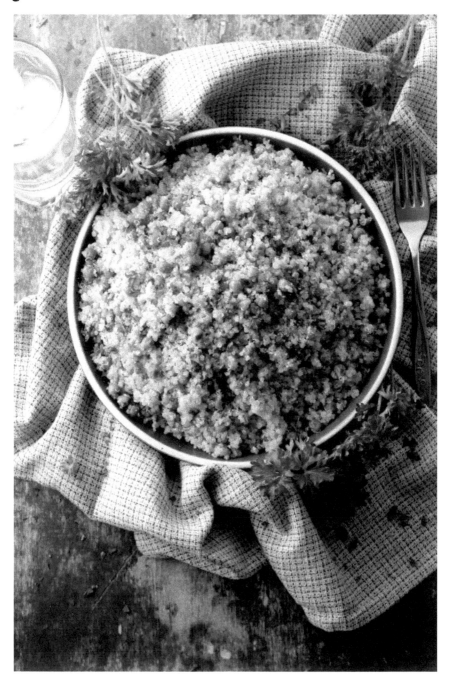

Preparation time: 10 minutes Cooking time: 30 minutes Servings: 4

Ingredients:

1 yellow onion, chopped

1 tomato, cubed

1 cup quinoa

3 cups vegetable stock

1 tablespoon olive oil

1 cup peas

1 tablespoon cilantro, chopped

A pinch of salt and black pepper

Directions:

1.   Heat up a pot with the oil over medium heat, add the onion, stir and sauté for 5 minutes.

2.   Add the quinoa, the stock and the other ingredients, toss, bring to a simmer and cook over medium heat for 25 minutes.

3.   Divide everything between plates and serve as a side dish.

Nutrition: calories 202, fat 3, fiber 3, carbs 11, protein 6

Basil Green Beans

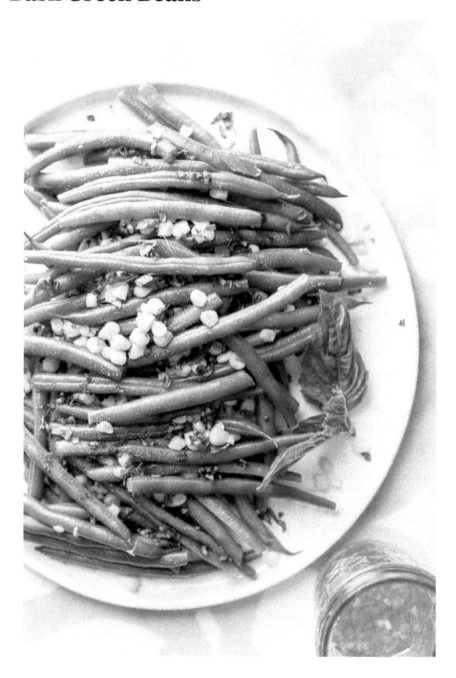

Preparation time: 10 minutes Cooking time: 20 minutes Servings: 4

Ingredients:

1 yellow onion, chopped

1-pound green beans, trimmed and halved

1 tablespoon avocado oil

2   teaspoons basil, dried

A pinch of salt and black pepper

1 tablespoon tomato sauce

Directions:

1.   Heat up a pan with the oil over medium-high heat, add the onion and sauté for 5 minutes.

2.   Add the green beans and the other ingredients, toss, cook for 15 minutes more.

3.   Divide everything between plates and serve as a side dish.

Nutrition: calories 221, fat 5, fiber 8, carbs 10, protein 8

Balsamic Brussels Sprouts

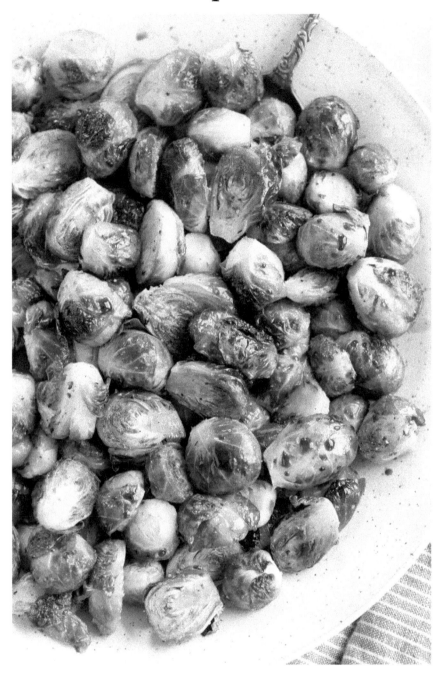

Preparation time: 10 minutes Cooking time: 20 minutes Servings: 4

Ingredients:

2 pounds Brussels sprouts, trimmed and halved

1 tablespoon avocado oil

2 tablespoons balsamic vinegar

3 garlic cloves, minced

1 tablespoon cilantro, chopped

A pinch of salt and black pepper

Directions:

1.   Heat up a pan with the oil over medium-high heat, add the garlic and sauté for 2 minutes.

2.   Add the sprouts and the other ingredients, toss, cook over medium heat for 18 minutes more, divide between plates and serve.

Nutrition: calories 108, fat 1.2, fiber 8.7, carbs 21.7, protein 7.9

Beet and Cabbage

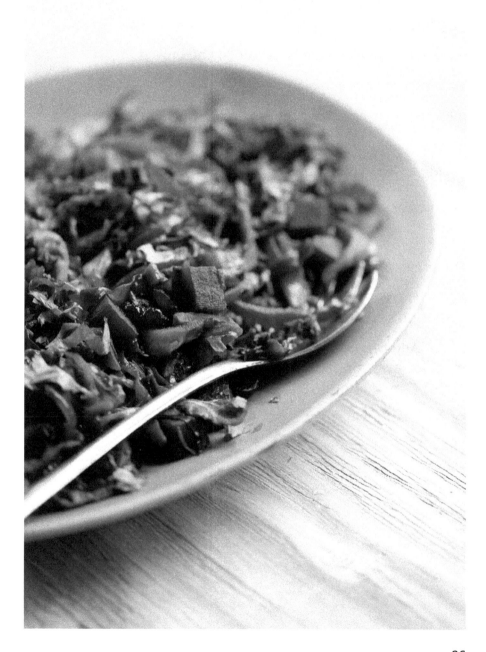

Preparation time: 10 minutes

Cooking time: 20 minutes Servings: 4

Ingredients:

1 green cabbage head, shredded

1 yellow onion, chopped

1 beet, peeled and cubed

½ cup chicken stock

2 tablespoons olive oil

A pinch of salt and black pepper

2 tablespoons chives, chopped

Directions:

1.   Heat up a pan with the oil over medium heat, add the onion and sauté for 5 minutes.

2.   Add the cabbage and the other ingredients, toss, cook over medium heat for 15 minutes more, divide between plates and serve.

Nutrition: calories 128, fat 7.3, fiber 5.6, carbs 15.6, protein 3.1

Chili Asparagus

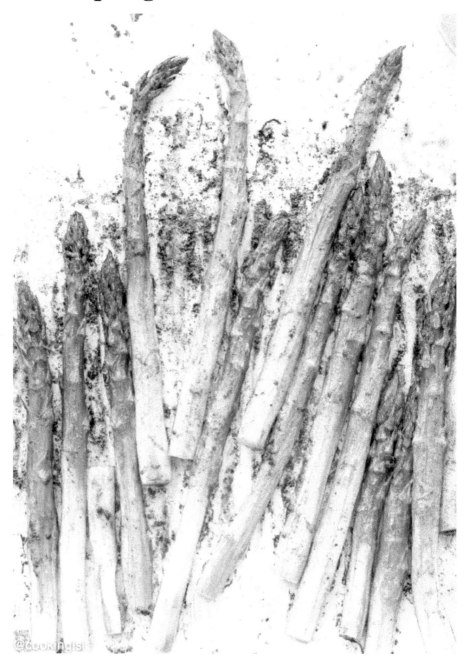

Preparation time: 10 minutes Cooking time: 15 minutes Servings: 4

Ingredients:

1 yellow onion, chopped

2 tablespoons olive oil

1 bunch asparagus, trimmed and halved

2 garlic cloves, minced

1 teaspoon chili powder

¼ cup cilantro, chopped

Directions:

1.   Heat up a pan with the oil over medium-high heat, add the onion and the garlic and sauté for 5 minutes.

2.   Add the asparagus and the other ingredients, toss, cook for 10 minutes, divide between plates and serve.

Nutrition: calories 80, fat 7.2, fiber 1.4, carbs 4.4, protein 1

Tomato Quinoa

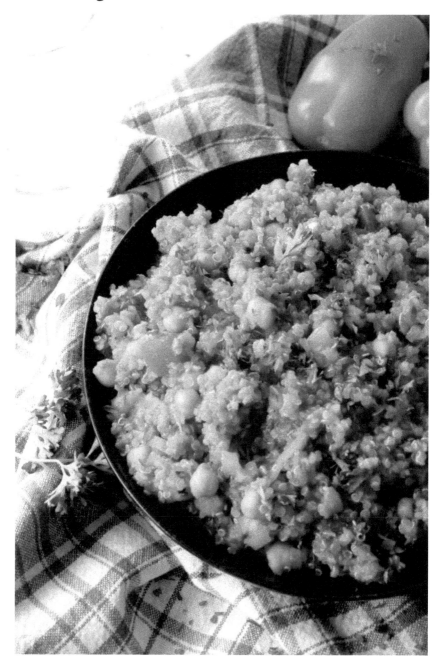

Preparation time: 10 minutes Cooking time: 25 minutes Servings: 4

Ingredients:

1 cup quinoa

3 cups chicken stock

1 cup tomatoes, cubed

1 tablespoon parsley, chopped

1 tablespoon basil, chopped

1 teaspoon turmeric powder

A pinch of salt and black pepper

Directions:

1. In a pot, mix the quinoa with the stock, the tomatoes and the other ingredients, toss, bring to a simmer and cook over medium heat for 25 minutes.

2. Divide everything between plates and serve.

Nutrition: calories 202, fat 4, fiber 2, carbs 12, protein 10

Coriander Black Beans

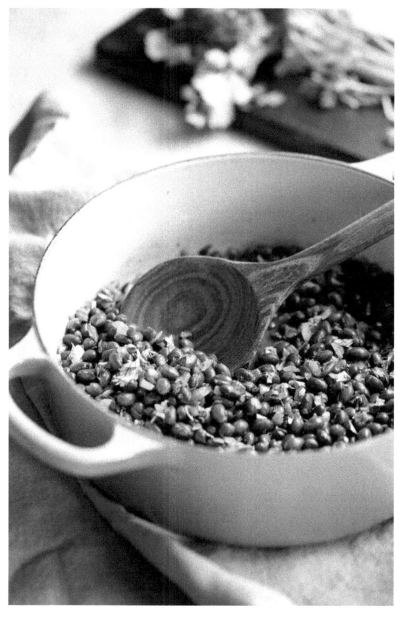

Preparation time: 10 minutes Cooking time: 20 minutes Servings: 4

Ingredients:

1   tablespoon olive oil

2   cups canned black beans, drained and rinsed

1 green bell pepper, chopped

1 yellow onion, chopped

4 garlic cloves, minced

1 teaspoon cumin, ground

½ cup chicken stock

1 tablespoon coriander, chopped

A pinch of salt and black pepper

Directions:

1.   Heat up a pan with the oil over medium heat, add the onion and the garlic and sauté for 5 minutes.

2.   Add the black beans and the other ingredients, toss, cook over medium heat for 15 minutes more, divide between plates and serve.

Nutrition: calories 221, fat 5, fiber 4, carbs 9, protein 11

Green Beans and Mango Mix

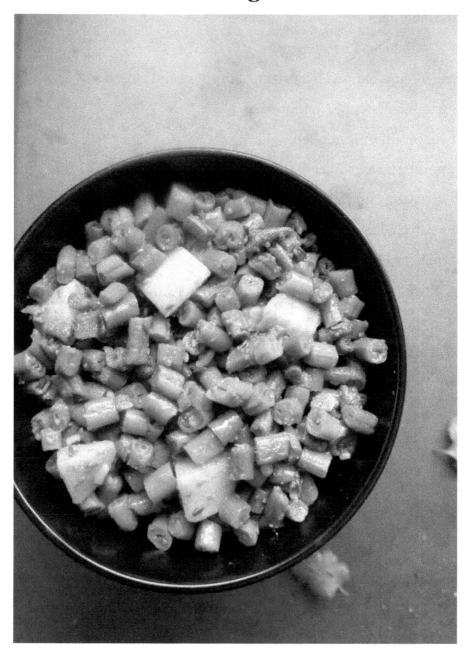

Preparation time: 10 minutes Cooking time: 20 minutes Servings: 4

Ingredients:

1 pound green beans, trimmed and halved

3 scallions, chopped

1 mango, peeled and cubed

2 tablespoons olive oil

½ cup veggie stock

1 tablespoon oregano, chopped

1 teaspoon sweet paprika

A pinch of salt and black pepper

Directions:

1.   Heat up a pan with the oil over medium heat, add the scallions and sauté for 2 minutes.

2.   Add the green beans and the other ingredients, toss, cook over medium heat for 18 minutes more, divide between plates and serve.

Nutrition: calories 182, fat 4, fiber 5, carbs 6, protein 8

Quinoa with Olives

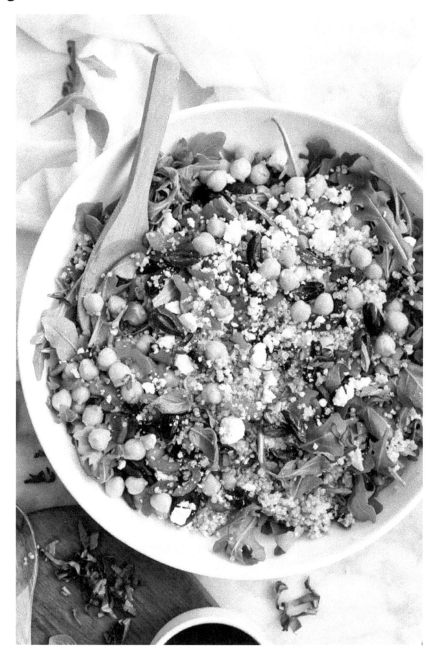

Preparation time: 10 minutes Cooking time: 30 minutes Servings: 4

Ingredients:

1 yellow onion, chopped

 tablespoon olive oil

1 cup quinoa

3 cups vegetable stock

½ cup black olives, pitted and halved

2 green onions, chopped

2 tablespoons coconut aminos

 1 teaspoon rosemary, dried

Directions:

1.   Heat up a pot with the oil over medium heat, add the yellow onion and sauté for 5 minutes.

2.   Add the quinoa and the other ingredients except the green onions, stir, bring to a simmer and cook over medium heat for 25 minutes.

3.   Divide the mix between plates, sprinkle the green onions on top and serve.

Nutrition: calories 261, fat 6, fiber 8, carbs 10, protein 6

Sweet Potato Mash

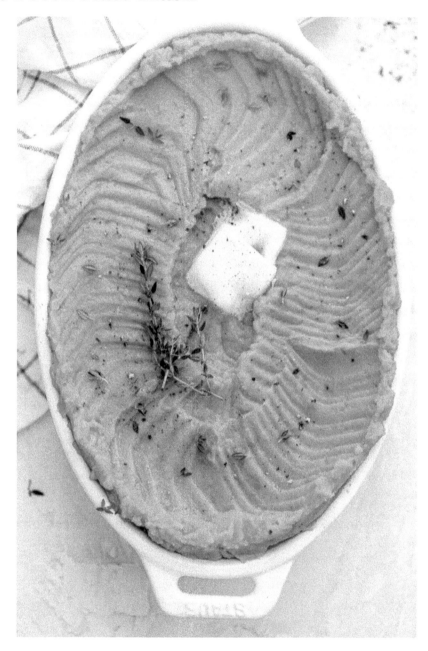

Preparation time: 10 minutes Cooking time: 25 minutes Servings: 4

Ingredients:

1 cup veggie stock

1 pound sweet potatoes, peeled and cubed

1 cup coconut cream

2   teaspoons olive oil

A pinch of salt and black pepper

½ teaspoon turmeric powder

1 tablespoon chives, chopped

Directions:

1.   In a pot, combine the stock with the sweet potatoes and the other ingredients except the cream, the oil and the chives, stir, bring to a simmer and cook over medium heat fro 25 minutes.

2.   Add the rest of the ingredients, mash the mix well, stir it, divide between plates and serve.

Nutrition: calories 200, fat 4, fiber 4, carbs 7, protein 10

Creamy Peas

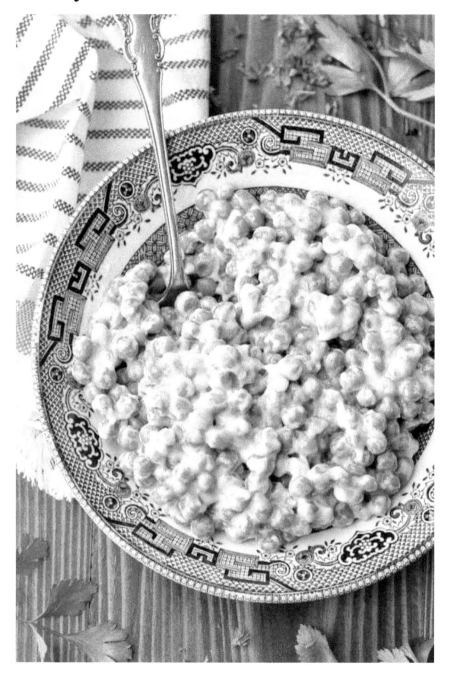

Preparation time: 10 minutes Cooking time: 20 minutes Servings: 4

Ingredients:

1 cup coconut cream

1   yellow onion, chopped

1 tablespoon olive oil

2   cups green peas

A pinch of salt and black pepper

A pinch of salt and black pepper

Directions:

1.   Heat up a pan with the oil over medium heat, add the onion and sauté for 5 minutes.

2.   Add the peas and the other ingredients, toss, cook over medium heat for 15 minutes, divide between plates and serve.

Nutrition: calories 191, fat 5, fiber 4, carbs 11, protein 9

Mushrooms and Black Beans

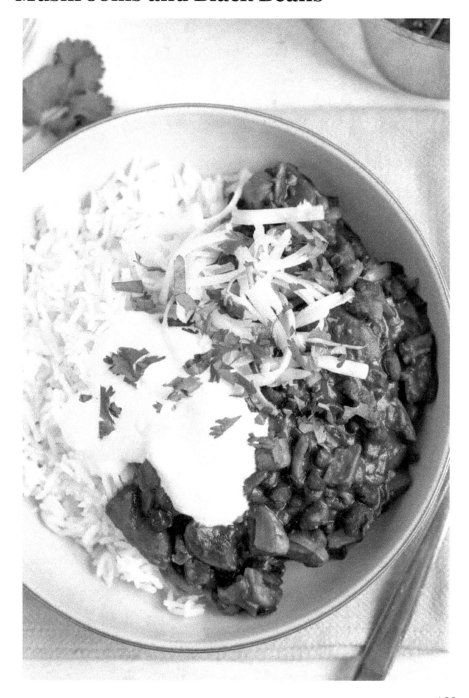

Preparation time: 10 minutes Cooking time: 25 minutes Servings: 4

Ingredients:

1 pound mushrooms, sliced

1 yellow onion, chopped

1 teaspoon cumin, ground

1 teaspoon sweet paprika

1 cup canned black beans, drained and rinsed

2 tablespoons olive oil

½ cup chicken stock

A pinch of salt and black pepper

2 tablespoons cilantro, chopped

Directions:

1.   Heat up a pan with the oil over medium heat, add the onion and sauté for 5 minutes.

2.   Add the mushrooms and sauté for 5 minutes more.

3.   Add the rest of the ingredients, toss, cook over medium heat for 15 minutes more.

4.   Divide everything between plates and serve as a side dish.

Nutrition: calories 189, fat 3, fiber 4, carbs 9, protein 8

Broccoli with Brussels Sprouts

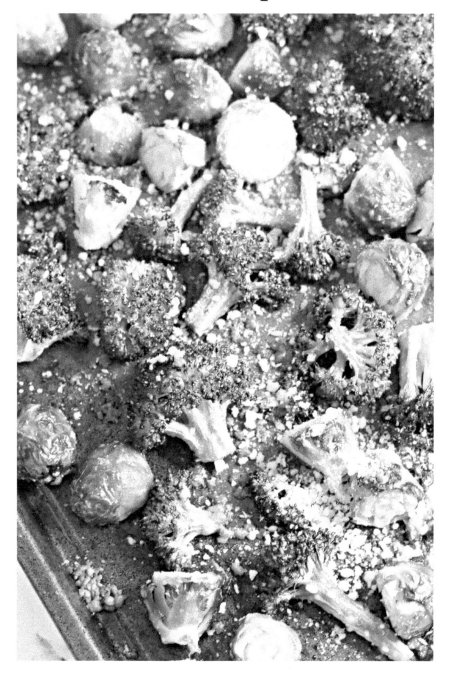

Preparation time: 10 minutes Cooking time: 25 minutes Servings: 4

Ingredients:

1 pound broccoli florets

½ pound Brussels sprouts, trimmed and halved

2 tablespoons olive oil

1 tablespoon ginger, grated

1 tablespoon balsamic vinegar

A pinch of salt and black pepper

Directions:

1.   In a roasting pan, combine the broccoli with the sprouts and the other ingredients, toss gently and bake at 380 degrees F for 25 minutes.

2.   Divide the mix between plates and serve.

Nutrition: calories 129, fat 7.6, fiber 5.3, carbs 13.7, protein 5.2

Glazed Cauliflower

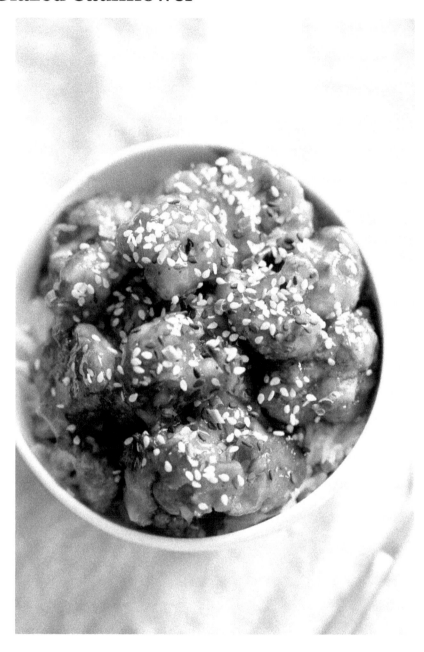

Preparation time: 10 minutes Cooking time: 25 minutes Servings: 4

Ingredients:

1 tablespoon olive oil

1 pound cauliflower florets 1 tablespoon maple syrup

1 tablespoon rosemary, chopped

A pinch of salt and black pepper 1 teaspoon chili powder

Directions

1.   Spread the cauliflower on a baking sheet lined with parchment paper, add the oil and the other ingredients, toss and cook in the oven at 375 degrees F for 25 minutes.

2.   Divide the mix between plates and serve.

Nutrition: calories 76, fat 3.9, fiber 3.4, carbs 10.3, protein 2.4

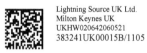

Lightning Source UK Ltd.
Milton Keynes UK
UKHW020642060521
383241UK00015B/1105